Easy

CALORIE DEFICIT COOKBOOK

Abibat Oladunjoye

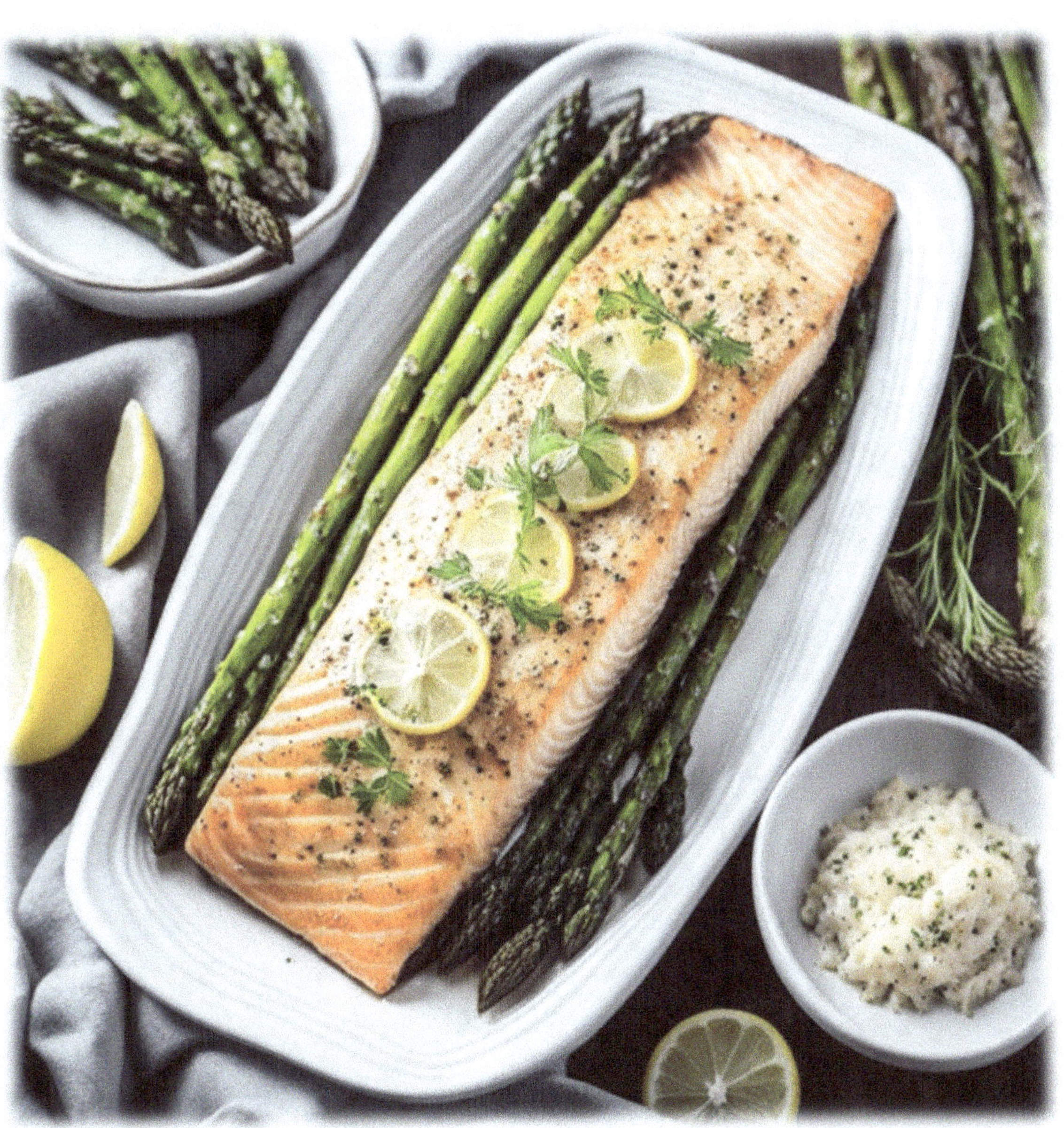

Contents

Introduction

Weight control ultimately boils down to one thing — calories. Despite all the diet strategies out there, weight management is fundamentally about the calories you consume versus those you burn off. Fad diets may promise that avoiding carbs or eating a mountain of grapefruit is the secret to weight loss, but it really comes down to eating fewer calories than your body uses if you want to shed pounds. Understanding this basic principle can help demystify weight loss and make it more attainable.

Reducing the amount of food you eat can be difficult in the long run, so this book provides a wealth of recipes and tips designed to help you maintain a calorie deficit without sacrificing flavor or satisfaction. The key is not to starve yourself but to make smarter food choices that keep you full and satisfied. Whether you are new to the concept of calorie counting or an experienced dieter looking for fresh ideas, this book has something for everyone. You'll find a variety of meals that are both delicious and nutritious, ensuring you never feel deprived while on your weight loss journey.

A balanced diet is crucial for maintaining overall health and well-being. It provides your body with the essential nutrients it needs to function correctly, support growth, and repair tissues. By focusing on a variety of foods that include all the major food groups, you can ensure that your body gets the vitamins, minerals, and energy it requires. This cookbook emphasizes the importance of balance by offering recipes that are not only low in calories but also rich in nutrients.

By combining delicious, satisfying meals with mindful eating, you can achieve your weight loss goals and maintain a healthy lifestyle. This book aims to make the process enjoyable and sustainable, providing you with the tools you need to succeed. Whether your goal is to lose weight, maintain your current weight, or simply eat healthier, these recipes are designed to support your journey.

1. Understanding Calories and Nutrition

What are Calories?

Definition and Importance

Calories are units of energy that fuel our bodies, much like gasoline powers a car. Every action, from thinking to running, requires energy, and that energy is measured in calories. Understanding the concept of calories is fundamental to managing weight and overall health.

How the Body Uses Calories

The body uses calories for three primary functions:

1. **Basal Metabolic Rate (BMR):** The energy needed for basic physiological functions, such as breathing, circulation, and cell production.
2. **Physical Activity:** The energy required for all forms of movement, from walking to intense exercise.
3. **Thermic Effect of Food (TEF):** The energy needed for digestion, absorption, and metabolism of food.

Macronutrients and Micronutrients

Carbohydrates, Proteins, and Fats

- **Carbohydrates:** The body's primary energy source, found in foods like grains, fruits, and vegetables. Carbs are essential for brain function and physical activity.
- **Proteins:** Crucial for building and repairing tissues, proteins are found in meats, dairy products, beans, and nuts. They play a key role in muscle maintenance and immune function.
- **Fats:** Necessary for absorbing vitamins and protecting organs, fats can be found in oils, butter, avocados, and nuts. While fats are calorie-dense, they are vital for overall health.

Vitamins and Minerals

- **Vitamins:** Organic compounds essential for various bodily functions. For example, vitamin C supports the immune system, while vitamin D promotes bone health.

- **Minerals:** Inorganic elements that play critical roles in the body. Calcium is essential for bones and teeth, while iron is crucial for oxygen transport in the blood.

Setting Your Calorie Goals

Calculating Basal Metabolic Rate (BMR)

Your BMR is the number of calories your body needs to maintain basic physiological functions at rest. Several formulas exist to calculate BMR, but a commonly used one is the Harris-Benedict Equation:

- For men: BMR = 88.362 + (13.397 × weight in kg) + (4.799 × height in cm) - (5.677 × age in years)
- For women: BMR = 447.593 + (9.247 × weight in kg) + (3.098 × height in cm) - (4.330 × age in years)

Determining Daily Calorie Needs

Once you have your BMR, multiply it by an activity factor to determine your Total Daily Energy Expenditure (TDEE):

- Sedentary (little or no exercise): BMR × 1.2

- Lightly active (light exercise/sports 1-3 days a week): BMR × 1.375

- Moderately active (moderate exercise/sports 3-5 days a week): BMR × 1.55

- Very active (hard exercise/sports 6-7 days a week): BMR × 1.725

- Super active (very hard exercise/sports and a physical job): BMR × 1.9

Setting a Safe and Effective Calorie Deficit

To lose weight, you need to create a calorie deficit by consuming fewer calories than your TDEE. A safe and sustainable calorie deficit is typically between 500-1000 calories per day, which can result in a weight loss of about 0.5-1 kg (1-2 pounds) per week. It's essential to avoid extreme calorie deficits, as they can lead to nutrient deficiencies, muscle loss, and other health issues.

2. Tools and Techniques for Healthy Cooking

Essential Kitchen Tools

To make healthy cooking easier and more enjoyable, it's important to have the right tools in your kitchen. Here are some must-have gadgets and utensils that will help you prepare delicious, low-calorie meals:

- **Knives:** A high-quality chef's knife, paring knife, and serrated knife are essential for efficient and precise cutting.
- **Cutting Boards:** Invest in a few cutting boards of different sizes, preferably made of wood or plastic, to keep your food preparation safe and organized.
- **Measuring Cups and Spoons:** Accurate measuring tools are crucial for portion control and following recipes correctly.
- **Mixing Bowls:** A set of mixing bowls in various sizes will help with preparing ingredients and mixing batters or salads.
- **Blender/Food Processor:** Perfect for smoothies, soups, sauces, and more, a good blender or food processor can save time and enhance the texture of your dishes.
- **Non-Stick Cookware:** Non-stick pans and pots require less oil for cooking, making it easier to prepare low-calorie meals.
- **Steamer Basket:** A steamer basket allows you to cook vegetables and other ingredients without added fat, preserving nutrients and flavor.
- **Baking Sheets and Pans:** Essential for roasting, baking, and more, these tools help you create a variety of healthy meals.
- **Spatulas and Tongs:** These utensils are useful for flipping, stirring, and serving food without adding extra calories from oil or butter.
- **Digital Kitchen Scale:** A scale helps you measure portions accurately, ensuring you stay within your calorie goals.

Cooking Methods

Choosing the right cooking methods can significantly impact the nutritional value and calorie content of your meals. Here are some healthy cooking techniques to incorporate into your kitchen routine:

- **Grilling:** Grilling meats, vegetables, and fruits enhances flavor without adding extra fat. Use a grill pan or an outdoor grill for best results.

- **Baking:** Baking is a versatile method that requires little to no added fat. Roast vegetables, bake fish, or prepare healthy casseroles in the oven.
- **Steaming:** Steaming preserves the nutrients in vegetables and other foods. Use a steamer basket or a dedicated steamer appliance for this method.
- **Sautéing:** Use a small amount of healthy oil, such as olive or avocado oil, to sauté vegetables, lean meats, and other ingredients quickly.
- **Slow Cooking:** A slow cooker is perfect for preparing soups, stews, and lean meats. This method allows flavors to meld while keeping calorie content low.
- **Poaching:** Cook foods gently in simmering water or broth. Poaching is ideal for eggs, fish, and chicken, adding flavor without extra calories.
- **Broiling:** Broiling uses high heat from above to cook food quickly, similar to grilling. It's great for finishing dishes with a crispy, browned top.

Healthy Ingredient Swaps

Making small changes to your ingredients can have a big impact on the calorie content and nutritional value of your meals. Here are some healthy swaps to consider:

- **Whole Grains for Refined Grains:** Use whole wheat pasta, brown rice, and whole grain bread instead of their refined counterparts to increase fiber and nutrients.
- **Greek Yogurt for Sour Cream or Mayonnaise:** Greek yogurt adds creaminess and protein with fewer calories.
- **Avocado for Butter or Margarine:** Use mashed avocado in baking or as a spread for a healthier fat option.
- **Zoodles for Pasta:** Substitute zucchini noodles (zoodles) for traditional pasta to cut carbs and calories.
- **Cauliflower for Rice or Potatoes:** Cauliflower rice and mashed cauliflower are lower-calorie alternatives to rice and mashed potatoes.
- **Spices and Herbs for Salt:** Enhance flavor with herbs and spices instead of relying on salt, which can contribute to high blood pressure.
- **Applesauce for Oil or Butter in Baking:** Applesauce adds moisture and sweetness with fewer calories and less fat.

Meal Prep Tips

Preparing meals in advance can save time, reduce stress, and help you stay on track with your calorie goals. Here are some tips for effective meal prep:

- **Plan Your Meals:** Decide on your meals and snacks for the week, and create a detailed shopping list.
- **Batch Cooking:** Cook large batches of staple ingredients like grains, proteins, and vegetables that can be mixed and matched throughout the week.
- **Use Proper Storage:** Invest in high-quality containers that are microwave and freezer-safe to keep your meals fresh and convenient to reheat.
- **Portion Control:** Divide meals into individual portions to avoid overeating and make it easier to grab a healthy meal on the go.
- **Label and Date:** Clearly label and date your prepped meals and ingredients to keep track of freshness and reduce food waste.
- **Incorporate Variety:** Prepare different recipes and ingredients to keep your meals interesting and prevent boredom.

3. Breakfast Recipes

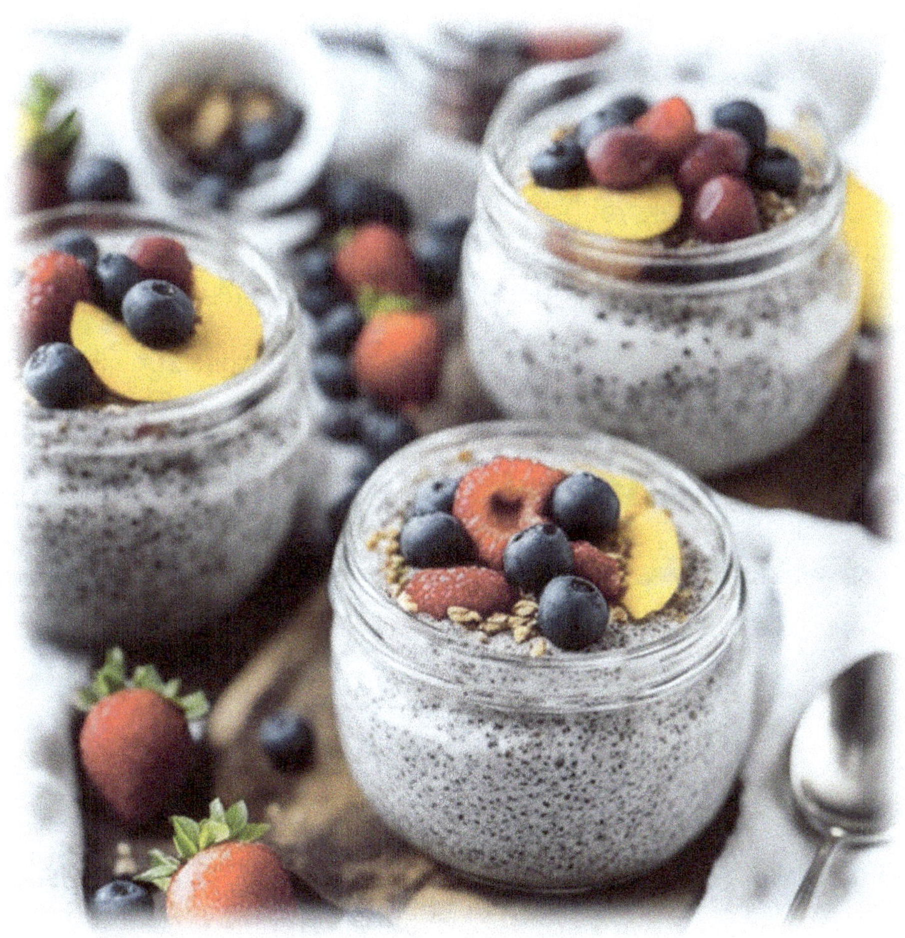

Greek Yogurt Parfait with Berries

Servings: 1

Cooking Time: 5 minutes

Ingredients

1 cup Greek yogurt (non-fat)

1/2 cup mixed berries (strawberries, blueberries, raspberries)

1 tablespoon honey

2 tablespoons granola

Instructions

1. Layer half of the Greek yogurt in a bowl or glass.
2. Add half of the mixed berries and drizzle with honey.
3. Add the remaining Greek yogurt, berries, and granola on top.

Nutritional Values: Calories: 220, Protein: 15g, Carbs: 30g, Fat: 4g

Spinach and Feta Egg White Omelette

Servings: 1

Cooking Time: 10 minutes

Ingredients:

4 egg whites

1/2 cup fresh spinach, chopped

1/4 cup feta cheese, crumbled

Salt and pepper to taste

Cooking spray or 1 tsp olive oil

Instructions

1. Spray a non-stick pan with cooking spray or heat olive oil over medium heat.
2. Add spinach and sauté until wilted.
3. Pour in the egg whites and cook until set, about 2-3 minutes.
4. Sprinkle feta cheese over half of the omelette and fold it in half. Season with salt and pepper.

Nutritional Values: Calories: 150, Protein: 20g, Carbs: 3g, Fat: 6g

Overnight Chia Pudding

Servings: 2

Cooking Time: 5 minutes (plus overnight refrigeration)

Ingredients

1/4 cup chia seeds

1 cup unsweetened almond milk

1 tablespoon maple syrup or honey

1/2 teaspoon vanilla extract

Fresh fruit for topping

Instructions

1. In a bowl, mix chia seeds, almond milk, maple syrup, and vanilla extract.
2. Stir well, cover, and refrigerate overnight.
3. Stir again in the morning and top with fresh fruit.

Nutritional Values: Calories: 180, Protein: 5g, Carbs: 22g, Fat: 9g

Avocado Toast on Whole Grain Bread

Servings: 1

Cooking Time: 5 minutes

Ingredients

1 slice whole grain bread, toasted

1/2 avocado, mashed

Salt and pepper to taste

Red pepper flakes (optional)

Instructions

1. Spread mashed avocado on toasted bread.
2. Season with salt, pepper, and red pepper flakes if desired.

Nutritional Values: Calories: 200, Protein: 5g, Carbs: 22g, Fat: 12g

Smoothie Bowl with Fresh Fruits and Nuts

Servings: 1

Cooking Time: 10 minutes

Ingredients

1/2 cup frozen berries

1/2 banana

1/2 cup Greek yogurt

1/4 cup almond milk

1 tablespoon chia seeds

1 tablespoon granola

Fresh fruit and nuts for topping

Instructions

1. Blend frozen berries, banana, Greek yogurt, almond milk, and chia seeds until smooth.
2. Pour into a bowl and top with granola, fresh fruit, and nuts.

Nutritional Values: Calories: 300, Protein: 12g, Carbs: 40g, Fat: 10g

Oatmeal with Almond Butter and Banana

Servings: 1

Cooking Time: 5 minutes

Ingredients

1/2 cup rolled oats

1 cup water or milk

1 tablespoon almond butter

1/2 banana, sliced

1 teaspoon honey (optional)

Instructions

1. Cook oats according to package instructions using water or milk.
2. Stir in almond butter and top with sliced banana and honey.

Nutritional Values: Calories: 250, Protein: 6g, Carbs: 40g, Fat: 10g

Vegetable and Cheese Breakfast Muffins

Servings: 6 muffins

Cooking Time: 30 minutes

Ingredients

6 large eggs

1/2 cup diced bell peppers

1/2 cup chopped spinach

1/4 cup shredded cheddar cheese

Salt and pepper to taste

Instructions

1. Preheat oven to 350°F (175°C) and grease a muffin tin.
2. In a bowl, whisk eggs and mix in vegetables, cheese, salt, and pepper.
3. Pour the mixture into the muffin tin, filling each cup about 3/4 full.
4. Bake for 20-25 minutes or until set.

Nutritional Values (per muffin): Calories: 100, Protein: 8g, Carbs: 2g, Fat: 7g

Berry and Spinach Smoothie

Servings: 1

Cooking Time: 5 minutes

Ingredients

1 cup spinach

1/2 cup frozen mixed berries

1/2 banana

1/2 cup Greek yogurt

1/2 cup water or almond milk

Instructions

1. Blend all ingredients until smooth.

Nutritional Values: Calories: 180, Protein: 10g, Carbs: 32g, Fat: 3g

Peanut Butter and Banana Rice Cakes

Servings: 1

Cooking Time: 5 minutes

Ingredients

2 brown rice cakes

1 tablespoon peanut butter

1/2 banana, sliced

Instructions

1. Spread peanut butter on rice cakes.
2. Top with banana slices.

Nutritional Values: Calories: 210, Protein: 5g, Carbs: 30g, Fat: 8g

Cottage Cheese and Fruit Bowl

Servings: 1

Cooking Time: 5 minutes

Ingredients

1 cup cottage cheese (low-fat)

1/2 cup mixed berries or other fruits

1 tablespoon honey

Instructions

1. In a bowl, combine cottage cheese and fruit.
2. Drizzle with honey.

Nutritional Values: Calories: 200, Protein: 20g, Carbs: 20g, Fat: 4g

Scrambled Tofu with Vegetables

Servings: 2

Cooking Time: 15 minutes

Ingredients

1 block firm tofu, drained and crumbled

1/2 cup diced bell peppers

1/2 cup chopped spinach

1/4 cup diced onions

1 tablespoon olive oil

1/2 teaspoon turmeric

Salt and pepper to taste

Instructions

1. Heat olive oil in a pan over medium heat.
2. Sauté onions and bell peppers until soft.
3. Add crumbled tofu, spinach, turmeric, salt, and pepper.
4. Cook for 5-7 minutes, stirring occasionally.

Nutritional Values: Calories: 200, Protein: 15g, Carbs: 10g, Fat: 10g

Apple Cinnamon Overnight Oats

Servings: 1

Cooking Time: 5 minutes (plus overnight refrigeration)

Ingredients

1/2 cup rolled oats

1/2 cup unsweetened almond milk

1/2 apple, diced

1 teaspoon cinnamon

1 teaspoon honey

Instructions

1. In a jar, combine oats, almond milk, apple, cinnamon, and honey.
2. Stir well, cover, and refrigerate overnight.

Nutritional Values: Calories: 220, Protein: 5g, Carbs: 40g, Fat: 5g

Turkey Sausage and Egg Breakfast Burrito

Servings: 1

Cooking Time: 10 minutes

Ingredients

1 whole wheat tortilla

2 egg whites

1 turkey sausage link, cooked and sliced

1/4 cup diced tomatoes

1 tablespoon shredded cheddar cheese

Salsa (optional)

Instructions

1. Cook egg whites in a non-stick pan.
2. Fill the tortilla with egg whites, turkey sausage, tomatoes, cheese, and salsa if desired.
3. Roll up and serve.

Nutritional Values: Calories: 250, Protein: 20g, Carbs: 25g, Fat: 8g

Pumpkin Spice Smoothie

Servings: 1

Cooking Time: 5 minutes

Ingredients

1/2 cup pumpkin puree

1/2 banana

1 cup unsweetened almond milk

1/2 teaspoon pumpkin pie spice

1 tablespoon maple syrup

Instructions

1. Blend all ingredients until smooth.

Nutritional Values: Calories: 160, Protein: 2g, Carbs: 35g, Fat: 2g

Quinoa Breakfast Bowl with Berries and Nuts

Servings: 1

Cooking Time: 15 minutes

Ingredients

1/2 cup cooked quinoa

1/4 cup Greek yogurt

1/4 cup mixed berries

1 tablespoon chopped nuts

1 teaspoon honey

Instructions

1. In a bowl, combine quinoa, Greek yogurt, berries, and nuts.
2. Drizzle with honey.

Nutritional Values: Calories: 230, Protein: 10g, Carbs: 35g, Fat: 8g

Cinnamon Apple Pancakes

Servings: 2

Cooking Time: 20 minutes

Ingredients

1 cup whole wheat flour

1 tablespoon baking powder

1 teaspoon cinnamon

1/2 cup unsweetened applesauce

1 cup unsweetened almond milk

1/2 apple, thinly sliced

Cooking spray or 1 tsp olive oil

Instructions

1. In a bowl, mix flour, baking powder, and cinnamon.
2. Add applesauce and almond milk, stirring until smooth.
3. Heat a pan with cooking spray or olive oil over medium heat.
4. Pour batter onto the pan and place apple slices on top.
5. Cook until bubbles form, then flip and cook until golden brown.

Nutritional Values (per serving): Calories: 200, Protein: 6g, Carbs: 35g, Fat: 4g

Egg and Avocado Breakfast Sandwich

Servings: 1

Cooking Time: 10 minutes

Ingredients

1 whole wheat English muffin, toasted

1 egg, cooked to preference

1/2 avocado, sliced

Salt and pepper to taste

Instructions

1. Place the cooked egg on one half of the toasted English muffin.
2. Top with avocado slices, salt, and pepper.
3. Place the other half of the muffin on top and serve.

Nutritional Values: Calories: 250, Protein: 10g, Carbs: 30g, Fat: 10g

Blueberry Almond Smoothie

Servings: 1

Cooking Time: 5 minutes

Ingredients

1/2 cup frozen blueberries

1/2 banana

1 cup unsweetened almond milk

1 tablespoon almond butter

Instructions

1. Blend all ingredients until smooth.

Nutritional Values: Calories: 200, Protein: 4g, Carbs: 30g, Fat: 8g

Vegetable and Hummus Breakfast Wrap

Servings: 1

Cooking Time: 10 minutes

Ingredients

1 whole wheat tortilla

2 tablespoons hummus

1/4 cup shredded carrots

1/4 cup sliced cucumber

1/4 cup baby spinach

Instructions

1. Spread hummus over the tortilla.
2. Layer with carrots, cucumber, and spinach.
3. Roll up and serve.

Nutritional Values: Calories: 200, Protein: 6g, Carbs: 30g, Fat: 7g

Protein-Packed Breakfast Bars

Servings: 6 bars

Cooking Time: 30 minutes

Ingredients

1 cup rolled oats

1/2 cup peanut butter

1/4 cup honey

1/2 cup protein powder (vanilla or chocolate)

1/4 cup unsweetened almond milk

1/4 cup dark chocolate chips (optional)

1. Preheat oven to 350°F (175°C) and line a baking dish with parchment paper.
2. In a bowl, mix oats, peanut butter, honey, protein powder, and almond milk.
3. Spread the mixture in the baking dish and sprinkle with chocolate chips if desired.
4. Bake for 15-20 minutes until set.
5. Let cool and cut into bars.

Nutritional Values (per bar): Calories: 250, Protein: 10g, Carbs: 30g, Fat: 10g

4. Lunch Recipes

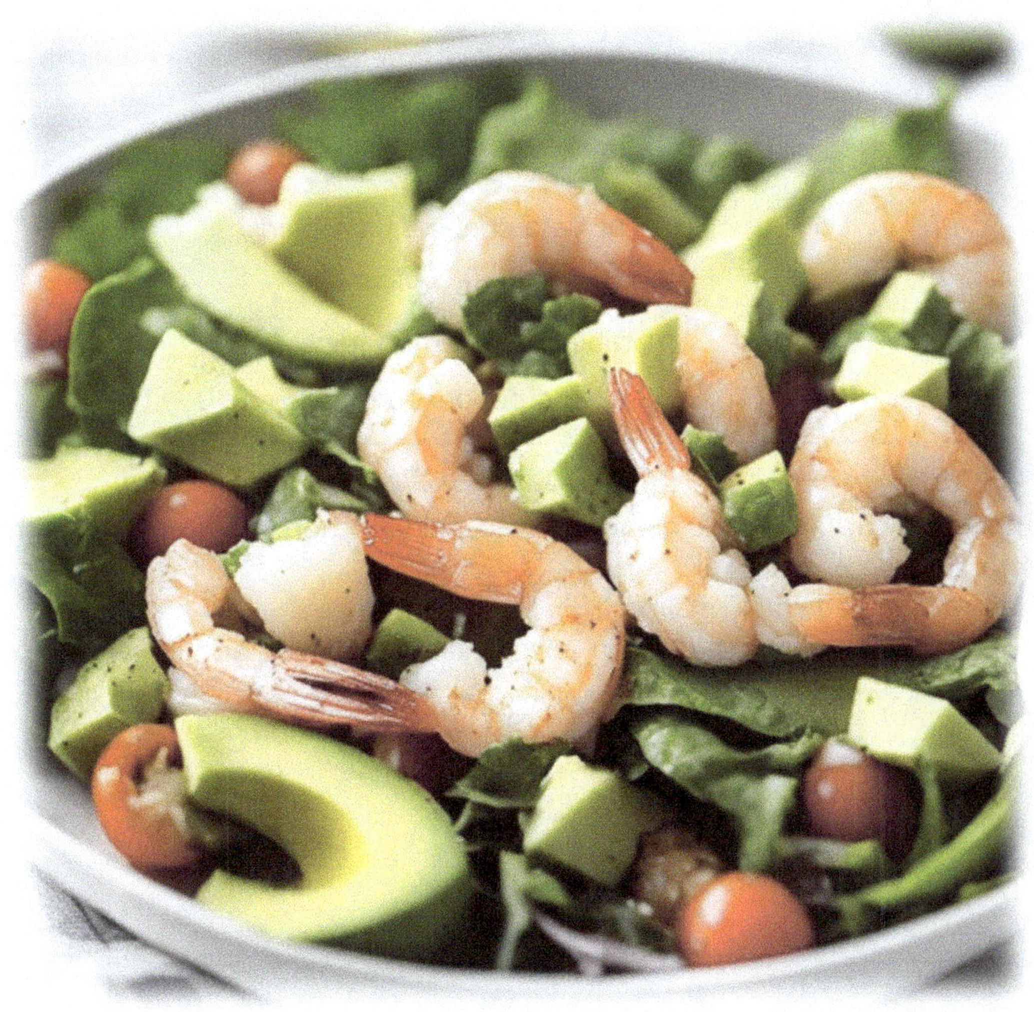

Grilled Chicken and Quinoa Salad

Servings: 2

Cooking Time: 30 minutes

Ingredients

1 cup cooked quinoa

1 chicken breast, grilled and sliced

1 cup mixed greens

1/2 cup cherry tomatoes, halved

1/4 cup cucumber, diced

1/4 cup feta cheese, crumbled

2 tablespoons olive oil

1 tablespoon lemon juice

Salt and pepper to taste

Instructions

1. In a large bowl, combine quinoa, mixed greens, cherry tomatoes, cucumber, and feta cheese.
2. Top with grilled chicken slices.
3. Drizzle with olive oil and lemon juice. Season with salt and pepper.

Nutritional Values: Calories: 350, Protein: 30g, Carbs: 30g, Fat: 14g

Turkey and Avocado Wrap

Servings: 1

Cooking Time: 10 minutes

Ingredients

1 whole wheat tortilla

4 slices turkey breast

1/2 avocado, sliced

1/4 cup baby spinach

1 tablespoon Greek yogurt

1 teaspoon Dijon mustard

Instructions

1. Spread Greek yogurt and Dijon mustard on the tortilla.
2. Layer turkey slices, avocado, and baby spinach.
3. Roll up the tortilla and slice in half.

Nutritional Values: Calories: 320, Protein: 25g, Carbs: 30g, Fat: 12g

Vegetable Stir-Fry with Tofu

Servings: 2

Cooking Time: 20 minutes

Ingredients

1 block firm tofu, cubed

2 cups mixed vegetables (bell peppers, broccoli, carrots)

2 tablespoons soy sauce

1 tablespoon olive oil

1 clove garlic, minced

1 teaspoon ginger, grated

1/2 cup brown rice, cooked

Instructions

1. Heat olive oil in a pan over medium heat.
2. Add garlic and ginger, sauté for 1 minute.
3. Add tofu and cook until golden brown.
4. Add mixed vegetables and soy sauce, stir-fry until vegetables are tender.
5. Serve over brown rice.

Nutritional Values: Calories: 350, Protein: 15g, Carbs: 40g, Fat: 15g

Lentil Soup

Servings: 4

Cooking Time: 45 minutes

Ingredients

1 cup lentils, rinsed

1 onion, diced

2 carrots, diced

2 celery stalks, diced

2 cloves garlic, minced

1 can diced tomatoes (14.5 oz)

4 cups vegetable broth

1 teaspoon cumin

1 teaspoon paprika

Salt and pepper to taste

Instructions

1. In a large pot, sauté onions, carrots, celery, and garlic until soft.
2. Add lentils, diced tomatoes, vegetable broth, cumin, and paprika.
3. Bring to a boil, then simmer for 30 minutes or until lentils are tender.
4. Season with salt and pepper.

Nutritional Values: Calories: 250, Protein: 15g, Carbs: 40g, Fat: 3g

Tuna Salad Lettuce Wraps

Servings: 2

Cooking Time: 10 minutes

Ingredients

1 can tuna (5 oz), drained

1/4 cup Greek yogurt

1 tablespoon lemon juice

1 celery stalk, diced

Salt and pepper to taste

4 large lettuce leaves

Instructions

1. In a bowl, mix tuna, Greek yogurt, lemon juice, and celery.
2. Season with salt and pepper.
3. Spoon the mixture onto lettuce leaves and roll up.

Nutritional Values: Calories: 200, Protein: 25g, Carbs: 5g, Fat: 8g

Chickpea and Spinach Salad

Servings: 2

Cooking Time: 15 minutes

Ingredients

1 can chickpeas (15 oz), drained and rinsed

2 cups baby spinach

1/4 cup red onion, thinly sliced

1/4 cup feta cheese, crumbled

2 tablespoons olive oil

1 tablespoon balsamic vinegar

Salt and pepper to taste

Instructions

1. In a large bowl, combine chickpeas, spinach, red onion, and feta cheese.
2. Drizzle with olive oil and balsamic vinegar. Season with salt and pepper.
3. Toss to coat and serve.

Nutritional Values: Calories: 280, Protein: 12g, Carbs: 30g, Fat: 14g

Chicken and Veggie Buddha Bowl

Servings: 2

Cooking Time: 30 minutes

Ingredients

1 chicken breast, grilled and sliced

1/2 cup quinoa, cooked

1/2 cup roasted sweet potatoes

1/2 cup steamed broccoli

1/4 avocado, sliced

2 tablespoons hummus

1 tablespoon lemon juice

Instructions

1. In a bowl, arrange quinoa, sweet potatoes, broccoli, avocado, and chicken slices.
2. Top with hummus and drizzle with lemon juice.

Nutritional Values: Calories: 400, Protein: 30g, Carbs: 45g, Fat: 14g

Caprese Sandwich

Servings: 1

Cooking Time: 10 minutes

Ingredients

2 slices whole grain bread

1/2 cup sliced fresh mozzarella

1/2 cup sliced tomatoes

1/4 cup fresh basil leaves

1 tablespoon balsamic glaze

Instructions

1. Layer mozzarella, tomatoes, and basil on one slice of bread.
2. Drizzle with balsamic glaze and top with the second slice of bread.

Nutritional Values: Calories: 320, Protein: 15g, Carbs: 40g, Fat: 12g

Black Bean and Corn Salad

Servings: 2

Cooking Time: 15 minutes

Ingredients

1 can black beans (15 oz), drained and rinsed

1 cup corn kernels

1/2 cup diced red bell pepper

1/4 cup red onion, diced

2 tablespoons lime juice

2 tablespoons olive oil

Salt and pepper to taste

Instructions

1. In a large bowl, combine black beans, corn, bell pepper, and red onion.
2. Drizzle with lime juice and olive oil. Season with salt and pepper.
3. Toss to coat and serve.

Nutritional Values: Calories: 300, Protein: 10g, Carbs: 45g, Fat: 10g

Miso Soup with Tofu and Seaweed

Servings: 2

Cooking Time: 15 minutes

Ingredients

4 cups water

2 tablespoons miso paste

1/2 block firm tofu, cubed

1/4 cup dried seaweed

2 green onions, sliced

Instructions

1. Bring water to a boil in a pot.
2. Add miso paste and stir until dissolved.
3. Add tofu and seaweed, simmer for 5 minutes.
4. Garnish with green onions and serve.

Nutritional Values: Calories: 150, Protein: 10g, Carbs: 10g, Fat: 6g

Shrimp and Avocado Salad

Servings: 2

Cooking Time: 20 minutes

Ingredients

1/2 lb cooked shrimp

1 avocado, diced

2 cups mixed greens

1/4 cup red bell pepper, diced

2 tablespoons olive oil

1 tablespoon lime juice

Salt and pepper to taste

Instructions

1. In a large bowl, combine shrimp, avocado, mixed greens, and bell pepper.
2. Drizzle with olive oil and lime juice. Season with salt and pepper.
3. Toss to coat and serve.

Nutritional Values: Calories: 350, Protein: 25g, Carbs: 20g, Fat: 20g

Turkey and Veggie Stuffed Peppers

Servings: 2

Cooking Time: 40 minutes

Ingredients

2 bell peppers, halved and seeded

1/2 lb ground turkey

1 cup cooked brown rice

1/2 cup diced tomatoes

1/4 cup shredded cheddar cheese

1 teaspoon garlic powder

Salt and pepper to taste

Instructions

1. Preheat oven to 375°F (190°C).
2. In a pan, cook ground turkey until browned. Add diced tomatoes, garlic powder, salt, and pepper.
3. Mix in cooked brown rice.
4. Stuff bell pepper halves with the turkey mixture.
5. Top with shredded cheddar cheese and bake for 20-25 minutes.

Nutritional Values: Calories: 300, Protein: 25g, Carbs: 30g, Fat: 10g

Zucchini Noodles with Pesto

Servings: 2

Cooking Time: 15 minutes

Ingredients

2 medium zucchinis, spiralized

1/4 cup pesto sauce

1/4 cup cherry tomatoes, halved

2 tablespoons grated Parmesan cheese

Instructions

1. In a pan, sauté zucchini noodles until tender, about 5 minutes.
2. Toss with pesto sauce and cherry tomatoes.
3. Sprinkle with grated Parmesan cheese and serve.

Nutritional Values: Calories: 220, Protein: 8g, Carbs: 15g, Fat: 15g

Chicken and Mango Salad

Servings: 2

Cooking Time: 20 minutes

Ingredients

1 chicken breast, grilled and sliced

1 mango, diced

2 cups mixed greens

1/4 cup red onion, sliced

2 tablespoons olive oil

1 tablespoon lime juice

Salt and pepper to taste

Instructions

1. In a large bowl, combine mixed greens, mango, red onion, and grilled chicken.
2. Drizzle with olive oil and lime juice. Season with salt and pepper.
3. Toss to coat and serve.

Nutritional Values: Calories: 350, Protein: 25g, Carbs: 35g, Fat: 14g

Eggplant and Tomato Sandwich

Servings: 1

Cooking Time: 20 minutes

Ingredients

2 slices whole grain bread

1/2 cup roasted eggplant slices

1/2 cup tomato slices

1 tablespoon hummus

1/4 cup fresh basil leaves

Instructions

1. Spread hummus on one slice of bread.
2. Layer with roasted eggplant, tomato slices, and basil leaves.
3. Top with the second slice of bread and serve.

Nutritional Values: Calories: 280, Protein: 8g, Carbs: 40g, Fat: 10g

Greek Yogurt Chicken Salad

Servings: 2

Cooking Time: 15 minutes

Ingredients

1 chicken breast, cooked and diced

1/4 cup Greek yogurt

1/4 cup diced celery

1/4 cup diced red grapes

1 tablespoon chopped walnuts

Salt and pepper to taste

Instructions

1. In a bowl, mix chicken, Greek yogurt, celery, grapes, and walnuts.
2. Season with salt and pepper.
3. Serve on a bed of lettuce or with whole grain crackers.

Nutritional Values: Calories: 280, Protein: 25g, Carbs: 15g, Fat: 12g

Spicy Chickpea and Avocado Sandwich

Servings: 1

Cooking Time: 10 minutes

Ingredients

2 slices whole grain bread

1/2 avocado, mashed

1/2 cup chickpeas, mashed

1 teaspoon sriracha sauce

1/4 cup shredded carrots

Instructions

1. Mix mashed chickpeas with sriracha sauce.
2. Spread mashed avocado on one slice of bread.
3. Top with chickpea mixture and shredded carrots.
4. Place the other slice of bread on top and serve.

Nutritional Values: Calories: 300, Protein: 10g, Carbs: 40g, Fat: 12g

Quinoa and Black Bean Stuffed Peppers

Servings: 2

Cooking Time: 40 minutes

Ingredients

2 bell peppers, halved and seeded

1/2 cup cooked quinoa

1/2 cup black beans

1/4 cup corn kernels

1/4 cup diced tomatoes

1 teaspoon cumin

Salt and pepper to taste

1/4 cup shredded cheese (optional)

Instructions

1. Preheat oven to 375°F (190°C).
2. In a bowl, mix quinoa, black beans, corn, tomatoes, cumin, salt, and pepper.
3. Stuff bell pepper halves with the quinoa mixture.
4. Top with shredded cheese if desired.
5. Bake for 25-30 minutes.

Nutritional Values: Calories: 280, Protein: 10g, Carbs: 40g, Fat: 8g

Salmon and Avocado Salad

Servings: 2

Cooking Time: 20 minutes

Ingredients

1 salmon fillet, cooked and flaked

1 avocado, diced

2 cups mixed greens

1/4 cup cherry tomatoes, halved

2 tablespoons olive oil

1 tablespoon lemon juice

Salt and pepper to taste

Instructions

1. In a large bowl, combine mixed greens, avocado, cherry tomatoes, and flaked salmon.
2. Drizzle with olive oil and lemon juice. Season with salt and pepper.
3. Toss to coat and serve.

Nutritional Values: Calories: 350, Protein: 25g, Carbs: 15g, Fat: 24g

Sweet Potato and Black Bean Tacos

Servings: 2

Cooking Time: 30 minutes

Ingredients

1 sweet potato, diced and roasted

1 cup black beans, cooked

4 small corn tortillas

1/4 cup diced red onion

1/4 cup chopped cilantro

2 tablespoons lime juice

Salt and pepper to taste

Instructions

1. Preheat oven to 400°F (200°C). Roast diced sweet potato for 20 minutes or until tender.
2. Warm the tortillas in a pan or microwave.
3. Fill each tortilla with roasted sweet potatoes, black beans, red onion, and cilantro.
4. Drizzle with lime juice and season with salt and pepper.

Nutritional Values: Calories: 300, Protein: 10g, Carbs: 50g, Fat: 6g

5. Dinner Recipes

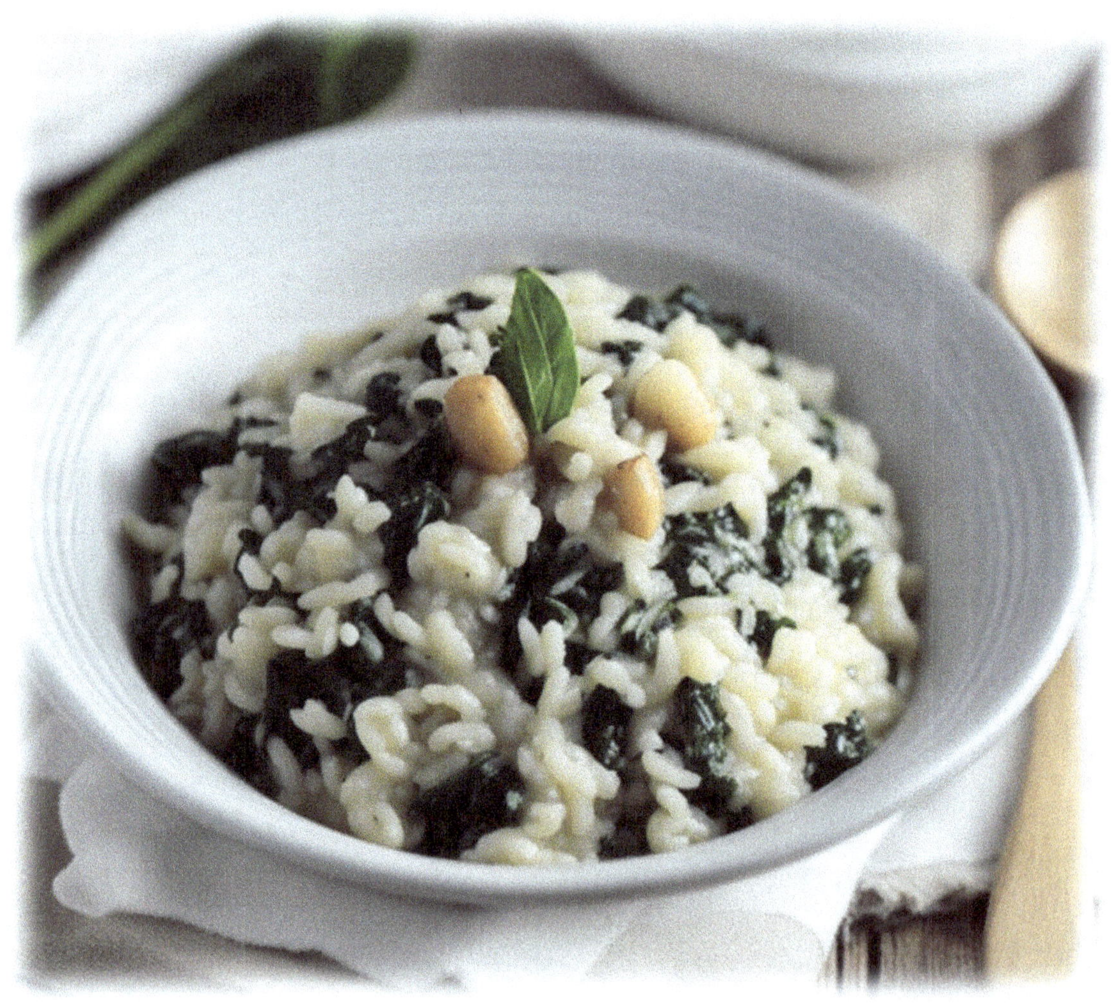

Baked Salmon with Asparagus

Servings: 2

Cooking Time: 25 minutes

Ingredients

2 salmon fillets

1 bunch asparagus, trimmed

2 tablespoons olive oil

1 tablespoon lemon juice

1 teaspoon garlic powder

Salt and pepper to taste

Instructions

1. Preheat oven to 400°F (200°C).
2. Place salmon fillets and asparagus on a baking sheet.
3. Drizzle with olive oil and lemon juice. Season with garlic powder, salt, and pepper.
4. Bake for 20 minutes or until salmon is cooked through.

Nutritional Values: Calories: 350, Protein: 30g, Carbs: 8g, Fat: 20g

Quinoa-Stuffed Bell Peppers

Servings: 4

Cooking Time: 40 minutes

Ingredients

4 bell peppers, halved and seeded

1 cup cooked quinoa

1 cup black beans, drained and rinsed

1 cup corn kernels

1 cup diced tomatoes

1 teaspoon cumin

Salt and pepper to taste

Instructions

1. Preheat oven to 375°F (190°C).
2. In a bowl, mix quinoa, black beans, corn, tomatoes, cumin, salt, and pepper.
3. Stuff bell pepper halves with the quinoa mixture.
4. Place in a baking dish and bake for 25-30 minutes.

Nutritional Values: Calories: 280, Protein: 10g, Carbs: 50g, Fat: 6g

Chicken and Broccoli Stir-Fry

Servings: 3

Cooking Time: 25 minutes

Ingredients

1 lb chicken breast, sliced

3 cups broccoli florets

1 bell pepper, sliced

2 tablespoons soy sauce

1 tablespoon olive oil

1 teaspoon ginger, grated

2 garlic cloves, minced

Instructions

1. Heat olive oil in a pan over medium heat.
2. Add garlic and ginger, sauté for 1 minute.
3. Add chicken and cook until no longer pink.
4. Add broccoli and bell pepper, stir-fry for 5 minutes.
5. Pour in soy sauce and cook for another 2-3 minutes.

Nutritional Values: Calories: 280, Protein: 30g, Carbs: 20g, Fat: 10g

Turkey Meatballs with Zucchini Noodles

Servings: 4

Cooking Time: 30 minutes

Ingredients

1 lb ground turkey

1 egg

1/4 cup breadcrumbs

2 tablespoons grated Parmesan cheese

2 garlic cloves, minced

1 teaspoon Italian seasoning

2 zucchinis, spiralized

1 cup marinara sauce

Instructions

1. Preheat oven to 375°F (190°C).
2. In a bowl, mix ground turkey, egg, breadcrumbs, Parmesan cheese, garlic, and Italian seasoning.
3. Form into meatballs and place on a baking sheet.
4. Bake for 20 minutes or until cooked through.
5. In a pan, heat marinara sauce and add zucchini noodles.
6. Serve meatballs over zucchini noodles.

Nutritional Values: Calories: 350, Protein: 35g, Carbs: 20g, Fat: 15g

Shrimp and Vegetable Skewers

Servings: 4

Cooking Time: 20 minutes

Ingredients

1 lb shrimp, peeled and deveined

1 red bell pepper, cut into chunks

1 yellow bell pepper, cut into chunks

1 zucchini, sliced

2 tablespoons olive oil

1 tablespoon lemon juice

1 teaspoon paprika

Salt and pepper to taste

Instructions

1. Preheat grill to medium-high heat.
2. Thread shrimp and vegetables onto skewers.
3. In a bowl, mix olive oil, lemon juice, paprika, salt, and pepper.
4. Brush skewers with the mixture.
5. Grill for 5-7 minutes on each side or until shrimp is cooked.

Nutritional Values: Calories: 250, Protein: 20g, Carbs: 15g, Fat: 10g

Lentil and Spinach Curry

Servings: 4

Cooking Time: 40 minutes

Ingredients

1 cup lentils, rinsed

4 cups spinach, chopped

1 onion, diced

2 tomatoes, diced

2 garlic cloves, minced

1 tablespoon curry powder

1 teaspoon cumin

1 teaspoon turmeric

2 cups vegetable broth

Instructions

1. In a pot, sauté onion and garlic until soft.
2. Add curry powder, cumin, and turmeric, cook for 1 minute.
3. Add lentils, tomatoes, and vegetable broth. Bring to a boil.
4. Reduce heat and simmer for 30 minutes or until lentils are tender.
5. Stir in spinach and cook until wilted.

Nutritional Values: Calories: 300, Protein: 15g, Carbs: 45g, Fat: 5g

Baked Cod with Lemon and Dill

Servings: 2

Cooking Time: 20 minutes

Ingredients

2 cod fillets

2 tablespoons olive oil

1 tablespoon lemon juice

1 teaspoon dried dill

Salt and pepper to taste

Instructions

1. Preheat oven to 400°F (200°C).
2. Place cod fillets on a baking sheet.
3. Drizzle with olive oil and lemon juice. Season with dill, salt, and pepper.
4. Bake for 15-20 minutes or until fish is cooked through.

Nutritional Values: Calories: 220, Protein: 30g, Carbs: 0g, Fat: 10g

Beef and Vegetable Stir-Fry

Servings: 4

Cooking Time: 25 minutes

Ingredients

1 lb beef sirloin, sliced

2 cups broccoli florets

1 bell pepper, sliced

1 carrot, sliced

2 tablespoons soy sauce

1 tablespoon olive oil

1 teaspoon ginger, grated

2 garlic cloves, minced

Instructions

1. Heat olive oil in a pan over medium heat.
2. Add garlic and ginger, sauté for 1 minute.
3. Add beef and cook until browned.
4. Add broccoli, bell pepper, and carrot, stir-fry for 5-7 minutes.
5. Pour in soy sauce and cook for another 2-3 minutes.

Nutritional Values: Calories: 350, Protein: 30g, Carbs: 15g, Fat: 20g

Spaghetti Squash with Tomato Sauce

Servings: 2

Cooking Time: 45 minutes

Ingredients

1 spaghetti squash

2 cups marinara sauce

1/4 cup grated Parmesan cheese

2 tablespoons olive oil

1 teaspoon Italian seasoning

Salt and pepper to taste

Instructions

1. Preheat oven to 375°F (190°C).
2. Cut spaghetti squash in half and remove seeds.
3. Drizzle with olive oil and season with salt and pepper.
4. Bake for 40 minutes or until tender.
5. Scrape the flesh with a fork to create strands.
6. Top with marinara sauce and Parmesan cheese.

Nutritional Values: Calories: 250, Protein: 10g, Carbs: 40g, Fat: 10g

Thai Peanut Chicken

Servings: 4

Cooking Time: 30 minutes

Ingredients

1 lb chicken breast, sliced

1 cup snap peas

1 red bell pepper, sliced

1/4 cup peanut butter

2 tablespoons soy sauce

1 tablespoon lime juice

1 teaspoon ginger, grated

2 garlic cloves, minced

Instructions

1. In a pan, cook chicken until no longer pink.
2. Add snap peas and bell pepper, cook for 5 minutes.
3. In a bowl, mix peanut butter, soy sauce, lime juice, ginger, and garlic.
4. Pour sauce over chicken and vegetables, cook for another 5 minutes.

Nutritional Values: Calories: 400, Protein: 30g, Carbs: 20g, Fat: 20g

Cauliflower Fried Rice

Servings: 4

Cooking Time: 20 minutes

Ingredients

1 head cauliflower, grated into rice-sized pieces

1 cup peas and carrots

2 eggs, beaten

2 tablespoons soy sauce

1 tablespoon sesame oil

2 garlic cloves, minced

Instructions

1. Heat sesame oil in a pan over medium heat.
2. Add garlic and cook for 1 minute.
3. Add peas and carrots, cook for 3-4 minutes.
4. Push vegetables to the side and pour beaten eggs into the pan, scramble until cooked.
5. Add grated cauliflower and soy sauce, cook for another 5-7 minutes.

Nutritional Values: Calories: 200, Protein: 10g, Carbs: 15g, Fat: 10g

Baked Chicken Parmesan

Servings: 4

Cooking Time: 30 minutes

Ingredients

4 chicken breasts

1 cup marinara sauce

1/2 cup shredded mozzarella cheese

1/4 cup grated Parmesan cheese

1 cup breadcrumbs

1 egg, beaten

Instructions

1. Preheat oven to 375°F (190°C).
2. Dip chicken breasts in beaten egg, then coat with breadcrumbs.
3. Place in a baking dish and bake for 20 minutes.
4. Top with marinara sauce and cheeses, bake for another 10 minutes.

Nutritional Values: Calories: 400, Protein: 40g, Carbs: 30g, Fat: 15g

Turkey and Sweet Potato Chili

Servings: 4

Cooking Time: 40 minutes

Ingredients

1 lb ground turkey

1 large sweet potato, diced

1 can black beans, drained and rinsed

1 can diced tomatoes

1 onion, diced

2 garlic cloves, minced

1 tablespoon chili powder

1 teaspoon cumin

Salt and pepper to taste

Instructions

1. In a pot, cook ground turkey until no longer pink.
2. Add onion and garlic, cook until soft.
3. Add sweet potato, black beans, tomatoes, chili powder, cumin, salt, and pepper.
4. Simmer for 30 minutes or until sweet potato is tender.

Nutritional Values: Calories: 350, Protein: 30g, Carbs: 40g, Fat: 10g

Tofu and Vegetable Stir-Fry

Servings: 4

Cooking Time: 25 minutes

Ingredients

1 block tofu, cubed

2 cups broccoli florets

1 bell pepper, sliced

1 carrot, sliced

2 tablespoons soy sauce

1 tablespoon olive oil

1 teaspoon ginger, grated

2 garlic cloves, minced

Instructions

1. Heat olive oil in a pan over medium heat.
2. Add garlic and ginger, sauté for 1 minute.
3. Add tofu and cook until browned.
4. Add broccoli, bell pepper, and carrot, stir-fry for 5-7 minutes.
5. Pour in soy sauce and cook for another 2-3 minutes.

Nutritional Values: Calories: 250, Protein: 15g, Carbs: 20g, Fat: 12g

Lemon Garlic Shrimp Pasta

Servings: 4

Cooking Time: 20 minutes

Ingredients

8 oz whole wheat pasta

1 lb shrimp, peeled and deveined

2 tablespoons olive oil

2 garlic cloves, minced

1 tablespoon lemon juice

1/4 cup grated Parmesan cheese

Instructions

1. Cook pasta according to package instructions.
2. In a pan, heat olive oil and sauté garlic until fragrant.
3. Add shrimp and cook until pink.
4. Add cooked pasta, lemon juice, and Parmesan cheese, toss to combine.

Nutritional Values: Calories: 400, Protein: 30g, Carbs: 50g, Fat: 12g

Veggie-Packed Frittata

Servings: 4

Cooking Time: 30 minutes

Ingredients

6 eggs

1/2 cup milk

1 cup spinach, chopped

1/2 cup bell pepper, diced

1/2 cup mushrooms, sliced

1/4 cup shredded cheese

Salt and pepper to taste

Instructions

1. Preheat oven to 375°F (190°C).
2. In a bowl, whisk eggs and milk. Season with salt and pepper.
3. Stir in spinach, bell pepper, mushrooms, and cheese.
4. Pour into a greased baking dish and bake for 20-25 minutes.

Nutritional Values: Calories: 250, Protein: 15g, Carbs: 10g, Fat: 18g

Baked Tilapia with Herbs

Servings: 4

Cooking Time: 20 minutes

Ingredients

4 tilapia fillets

2 tablespoons olive oil

1 tablespoon lemon juice

1 teaspoon dried thyme

1 teaspoon dried rosemary

Salt and pepper to taste

Instructions

1. Preheat oven to 400°F (200°C).
2. Place tilapia fillets on a baking sheet.
3. Drizzle with olive oil and lemon juice. Season with thyme, rosemary, salt, and pepper.
4. Bake for 15-20 minutes or until fish is cooked through.

Nutritional Values: Calories: 200, Protein: 30g, Carbs: 0g, Fat: 10g

Mushroom and Spinach Risotto

Servings: 4

Cooking Time: 35 minutes

Ingredients

1 cup Arborio rice

4 cups vegetable broth

1 cup mushrooms, sliced

2 cups spinach, chopped

1/4 cup grated Parmesan cheese

1 onion, diced

2 garlic cloves, minced

2 tablespoons olive oil

Instructions

1. Heat olive oil in a pan and sauté onion and garlic until soft.
2. Add mushrooms and cook until browned.
3. Stir in Arborio rice and cook for 1-2 minutes.
4. Gradually add vegetable broth, stirring frequently, until rice is creamy and tender.
5. Stir in spinach and Parmesan cheese.

Nutritional Values: Calories: 350, Protein: 10g, Carbs: 55g, Fat: 10g

Chickpea and Vegetable Curry

Servings: 4

Cooking Time: 30 minutes

Ingredients

1 can chickpeas, drained and rinsed

1 cup cauliflower florets

1 cup diced tomatoes

1 cup coconut milk

1 onion, diced

2 garlic cloves, minced

1 tablespoon curry powder

1 teaspoon cumin

Salt and pepper to taste

Instructions

1. In a pot, sauté onion and garlic until soft.
2. Add curry powder and cumin, cook for 1 minute.
3. Add chickpeas, cauliflower, tomatoes, and coconut milk.

4. Simmer for 20-25 minutes or until vegetables are tender.

Nutritional Values: Calories: 300, Protein: 10g, Carbs: 40g, Fat: 12g

Greek Chicken Bowls

Servings: 4

Cooking Time: 25 minutes

Ingredients

1 lb chicken breast, sliced

2 cups cooked quinoa

1 cup cucumber, diced

1 cup cherry tomatoes, halved

1/2 cup red onion, diced

1/4 cup feta cheese, crumbled

2 tablespoons olive oil

1 tablespoon lemon juice

1 teaspoon dried oregano

Salt and pepper to taste

Instructions

1. In a pan, heat olive oil and cook chicken until no longer pink.
2. In a bowl, mix quinoa, cucumber, cherry tomatoes, red onion, and feta cheese.
3. Add cooked chicken and season with lemon juice, oregano, salt, and pepper.

Nutritional Values: Calories: 400, Protein: 35g, Carbs: 35g, Fat: 12g

6. **Snack Recipes**

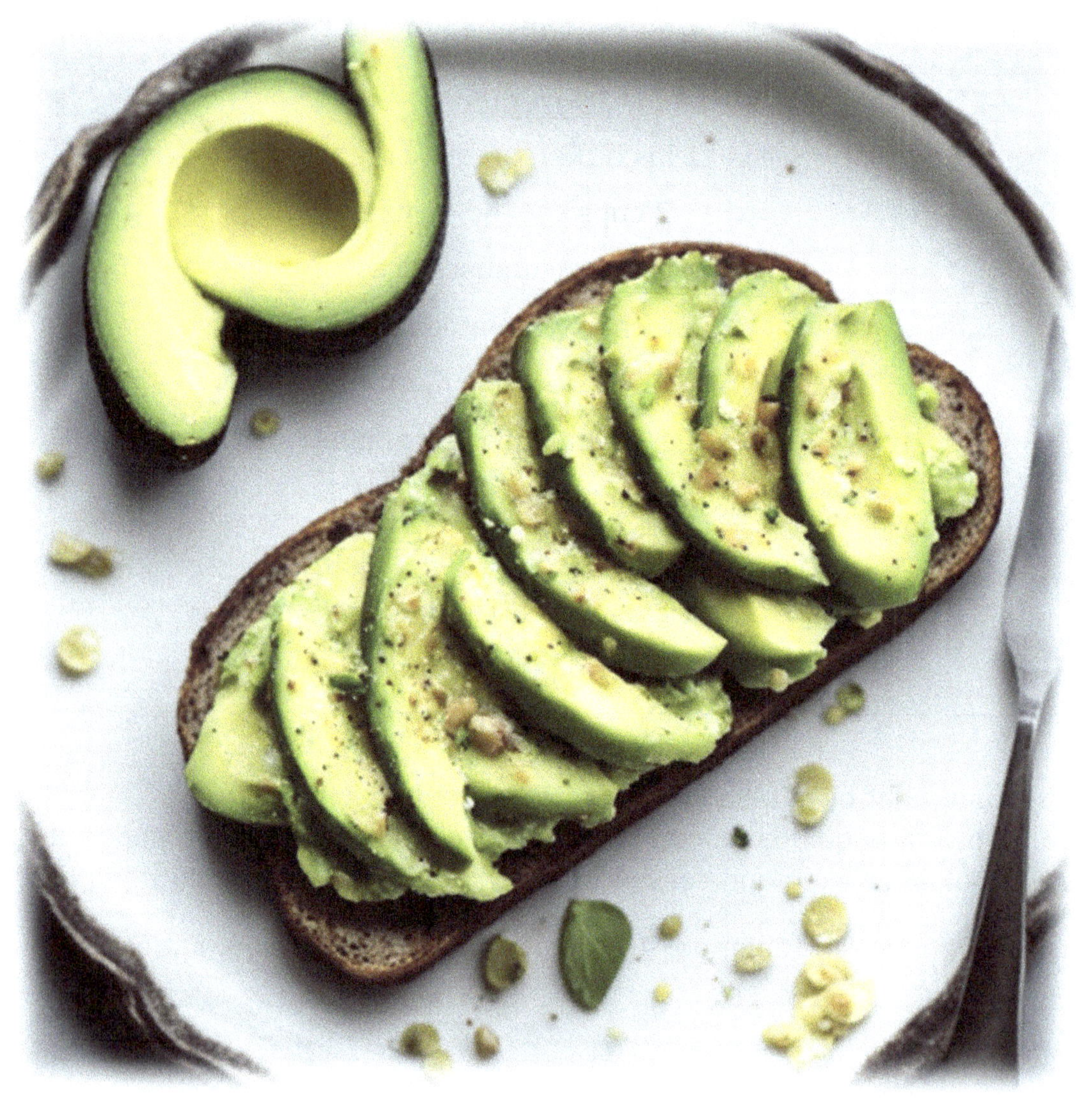

Greek Yogurt and Berry Parfait

Servings: 2

Cooking Time: 5 minutes

Ingredients

1 cup Greek yogurt

1/2 cup mixed berries (blueberries, strawberries, raspberries)

1 tablespoon honey

2 tablespoons granola

Instructions

1. Layer Greek yogurt, mixed berries, and honey in two cups.
2. Top with granola.

Nutritional Values: Calories: 200, Protein: 10g, Carbs: 30g, Fat: 4g

Hummus and Veggie Sticks

Servings: 2

Cooking Time: 10 minutes

Ingredients

1 cup hummus

1 carrot, cut into sticks

1 cucumber, cut into sticks

1 bell pepper, cut into sticks

Instructions

1. Serve hummus in a bowl with veggie sticks on the side.

Nutritional Values: Calories: 180, Protein: 5g, Carbs: 20g, Fat: 10g

Apple Slices with Almond Butter

Servings: 2

Cooking Time: 5 minutes

Ingredients

1 apple, sliced

2 tablespoons almond butter

Instructions

1. Serve apple slices with almond butter on the side.

Nutritional Values: Calories: 150, Protein: 4g, Carbs: 20g, Fat: 8g

Cottage Cheese and Pineapple

Servings: 2

Cooking Time: 5 minutes

Ingredients

1 cup cottage cheese

1/2 cup pineapple chunks

Instructions

1. Mix cottage cheese with pineapple chunks.

Nutritional Values: Calories: 160, Protein: 14g, Carbs: 20g, Fat: 2g

Spiced Chickpeas

Servings: 4

Cooking Time: 30 minutes

Ingredients

1 can chickpeas, drained and rinsed

1 tablespoon olive oil

1 teaspoon paprika

1 teaspoon cumin

1/2 teaspoon salt

Instructions

1. Preheat oven to 400°F (200°C).
2. Toss chickpeas with olive oil, paprika, cumin, and salt.
3. Spread on a baking sheet and bake for 25-30 minutes, stirring occasionally.

Nutritional Values: Calories: 120, Protein: 5g, Carbs: 15g, Fat: 4g

Avocado Toast

Servings: 1

Cooking Time: 5 minutes

Ingredients

1 slice whole grain bread, toasted

1/2 avocado, mashed

Salt and pepper to taste

Optional: cherry tomatoes, red pepper flakes

Instructions

1. Spread mashed avocado on toast.
2. Season with salt and pepper.

3. Top with cherry tomatoes and red pepper flakes if desired.

Nutritional Values: Calories: 250, Protein: 6g, Carbs: 30g, Fat: 12g

Peanut Butter Banana Bites

Servings: 2

Cooking Time: 5 minutes

Ingredients

1 banana, sliced

2 tablespoons peanut butter

Instructions

1. Spread peanut butter between banana slices to create mini sandwiches.

Nutritional Values: Calories: 180, Protein: 4g, Carbs: 26g, Fat: 8g

Trail Mix

Servings: 4

Cooking Time: 5 minutes

Ingredients

1/2 cup almonds

1/2 cup walnuts

1/4 cup dried cranberries

1/4 cup dark chocolate chips

Instructions

1. Mix all ingredients in a bowl.

Nutritional Values: Calories: 220, Protein: 5g, Carbs: 18g, Fat: 15g

Veggie Roll-Ups

Servings: 2

Cooking Time: 10 minutes

Ingredients

2 whole wheat tortillas

1/4 cup hummus

1/2 cup spinach leaves

1/4 cup shredded carrots

1/4 cup cucumber slices

Instructions

1. Spread hummus on tortillas.
2. Layer with spinach, carrots, and cucumber.
3. Roll up and slice into bite-sized pieces.

Nutritional Values: Calories: 180, Protein: 6g, Carbs: 28g, Fat: 6g

Edamame

Servings: 2

Cooking Time: 5 minutes

Ingredients

1 cup edamame, steamed

Salt to taste

Instructions

1. Steam edamame and sprinkle with salt.

Nutritional Values: Calories: 120, Protein: 10g, Carbs: 10g, Fat: 5g

Chia Seed Pudding

Servings: 2

Cooking Time: 5 minutes + 2 hours chilling time

Ingredients

1/4 cup chia seeds

1 cup almond milk

1 tablespoon honey

1/2 teaspoon vanilla extract

Instructions

1. Mix chia seeds, almond milk, honey, and vanilla extract in a bowl.
2. Refrigerate for at least 2 hours, stirring occasionally.

Nutritional Values: Calories: 150, Protein: 4g, Carbs: 18g, Fat: 7g

Popcorn

Servings: 2

Cooking Time: 10 minutes

Ingredients

1/4 cup popcorn kernels

1 tablespoon olive oil

Salt to taste

Instructions

1. Heat olive oil in a pot over medium heat.
2. Add popcorn kernels and cover.
3. Shake pot occasionally until popping slows down.
4. Season with salt.

Nutritional Values: Calories: 100, Protein: 3g, Carbs: 20g, Fat: 3g

Cottage Cheese and Tomato Slices

Servings: 2

Cooking Time: 5 minutes

Ingredients

1 cup cottage cheese

1 large tomato, sliced

Salt and pepper to taste

Instructions

1. Serve cottage cheese with tomato slices.
2. Season with salt and pepper.

Nutritional Values: Calories: 160, Protein: 14g, Carbs: 8g, Fat: 6g

Frozen Yogurt Bark

Servings: 4

Cooking Time: 5 minutes + 2 hours freezing time

Ingredients

2 cups Greek yogurt

1/4 cup honey

1/2 cup mixed berries

1/4 cup granola

Instructions

1. Mix Greek yogurt and honey.
2. Spread on a baking sheet lined with parchment paper.
3. Sprinkle with mixed berries and granola.
4. Freeze for at least 2 hours.
5. Break into pieces before serving.

Mini Caprese Skewers

Servings: 4

Cooking Time: 10 minutes

Ingredients

20 cherry tomatoes

20 small mozzarella balls

Fresh basil leaves

2 tablespoons balsamic glaze

Instructions

1. Thread cherry tomatoes, mozzarella balls, and basil leaves onto skewers.
2. Drizzle with balsamic glaze.

Nutritional Values: Calories: 100, Protein: 5g, Carbs: 5g, Fat: 7g

7. Dessert Recipes

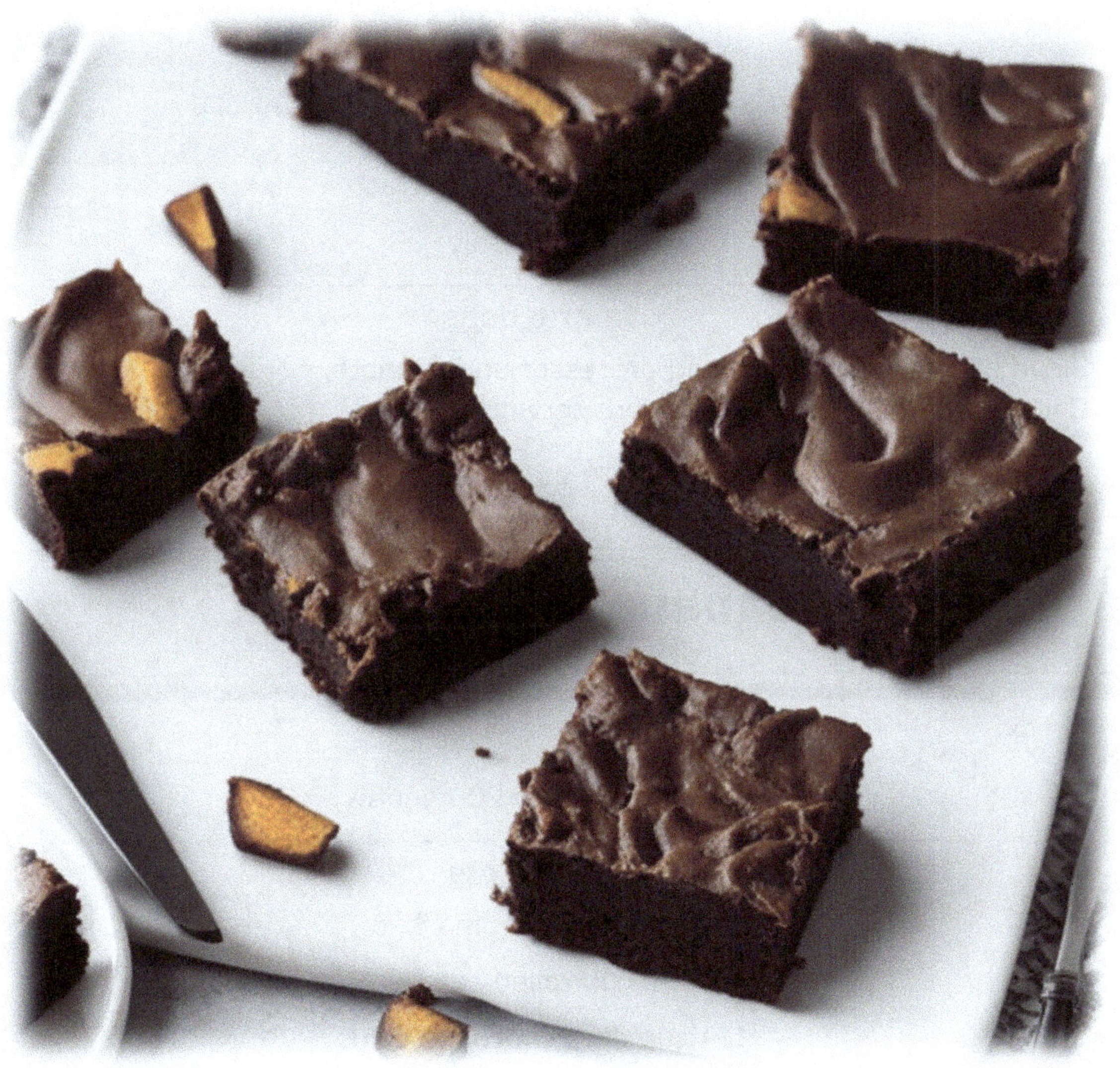

Chocolate Avocado Mousse

Servings: 4

Cooking Time: 10 minutes

Ingredients

2 ripe avocados

1/4 cup cocoa powder

1/4 cup honey

1 teaspoon vanilla extract

Pinch of salt

Instructions

1. Blend all ingredients in a food processor until smooth.
2. Chill for at least 30 minutes before serving.

Nutritional Values: Calories: 200, Protein: 2g, Carbs: 24g, Fat: 12g

Banana Oat Cookies

Servings: 12 cookies

Cooking Time: 20 minutes

Ingredients

2 ripe bananas, mashed

1 cup rolled oats

1/4 cup dark chocolate chips

1/4 cup chopped nuts (optional)

Instructions

1. Preheat oven to 350°F (175°C).
2. Mix all ingredients in a bowl.
3. Drop spoonfuls of dough onto a baking sheet.

4. Bake for 15-20 minutes or until golden brown.

Nutritional Values: Calories: 100, Protein: 2g, Carbs: 18g, Fat: 3g

Baked Apples with Cinnamon

Servings: 4

Cooking Time: 30 minutes

Ingredients

4 apples, cored

1/4 cup raisins

1 teaspoon cinnamon

1 tablespoon honey

1/4 cup chopped nuts (optional)

Instructions

1. Preheat oven to 375°F (190°C).
2. Stuff apples with raisins and nuts, sprinkle with cinnamon.
3. Drizzle with honey.
4. Bake for 25-30 minutes or until apples are tender.

Nutritional Values: Calories: 150, Protein: 1g, Carbs: 34g, Fat: 2g

Strawberry Chia Pudding

Servings: 2

Cooking Time: 5 minutes + 2 hours chilling time

Ingredients

1/4 cup chia seeds

1 cup almond milk

1/2 cup strawberries, mashed

1 tablespoon honey

1. Mix chia seeds, almond milk, mashed strawberries, and honey in a bowl.
2. Refrigerate for at least 2 hours, stirring occasionally.

Nutritional Values: Calories: 150, Protein: 4g, Carbs: 22g, Fat: 6g

Coconut Macaroons

Servings: 12

Cooking Time: 30 minutes

Ingredients

2 cups shredded coconut

1/2 cup sweetened condensed milk

1 teaspoon vanilla extract

Instructions

1. Preheat oven to 325°F (160°C).
2. Mix all ingredients in a bowl.
3. Drop spoonfuls of mixture onto a baking sheet.
4. Bake for 20-25 minutes or until golden brown.

Nutritional Values: Calories: 120, Protein: 1g, Carbs: 16g, Fat: 6g

Lemon Ricotta Cheesecake Bites

Servings: 12

Cooking Time: 25 minutes

Ingredients

1 cup ricotta cheese

2 tablespoons honey

1 tablespoon lemon zest

1 teaspoon vanilla extract

1. Preheat oven to 350°F (175°C).
2. Mix all ingredients until smooth.
3. Spoon mixture into mini muffin tin.
4. Bake for 20-25 minutes or until set.

Nutritional Values: Calories: 80, Protein: 4g, Carbs: 8g, Fat: 4g

Frozen Banana Bites

Servings: 4

Cooking Time: 5 minutes + 2 hours freezing time

Ingredients

2 bananas, sliced

1/4 cup dark chocolate chips, melted

1 tablespoon coconut oil

Instructions

1. Dip banana slices in melted chocolate mixed with coconut oil.
2. Place on a baking sheet lined with parchment paper.
3. Freeze for at least 2 hours.

Nutritional Values: Calories: 100, Protein: 1g, Carbs: 20g, Fat: 4g

Blueberry Muffins

Servings: 12 muffins

Cooking Time: 25 minutes

Ingredients

1 cup whole wheat flour

1/2 cup rolled oats

1/2 cup honey

1 teaspoon baking powder

1/2 teaspoon baking soda

1/2 teaspoon salt

1 cup blueberries

1/2 cup unsweetened applesauce

1 egg

1 teaspoon vanilla extract

Instructions

1. Preheat oven to 350°F (175°C).
2. Mix dry ingredients in a bowl.
3. In another bowl, mix wet ingredients.
4. Combine both mixtures and fold in blueberries.
5. Pour into muffin tin and bake for 20-25 minutes.

Nutritional Values: Calories: 120, Protein: 3g, Carbs: 25g, Fat: 2g

Mango Sorbet

Servings: 4

Cooking Time: 10 minutes + 2 hours freezing time

Ingredients

2 ripe mangoes, peeled and chopped

1/4 cup honey

1/2 cup water

Instructions

1. Blend all ingredients until smooth.
2. Pour into a container and freeze for at least 2 hours.

Nutritional Values: Calories: 100, Protein: 1g, Carbs: 26g, Fat: 0g

Almond Flour Brownies

Servings: 12 brownies

Cooking Time: 25 minutes

Ingredients

1 cup almond flour

1/2 cup cocoa powder

1/2 cup honey

1/4 cup coconut oil, melted

2 eggs

1 teaspoon vanilla extract

1/2 teaspoon baking powder

Instructions

1. Preheat oven to 350°F (175°C).
2. Mix all ingredients in a bowl until smooth.

3. Pour into a greased baking dish and bake for 20-25 minutes.

Nutritional Values: Calories: 140, Protein: 3g, Carbs: 16g, Fat: 8g

Sweet Potato Brownies

Servings: 12 brownies

Cooking Time: 30 minutes

Ingredients

1 cup mashed sweet potatoes

1/2 cup cocoa powder

1/4 cup maple syrup

1/4 cup almond butter

1/2 teaspoon baking powder

1/2 teaspoon vanilla extract

Instructions

1. Preheat oven to 350°F (175°C).
2. Mix all ingredients in a bowl until smooth.
3. Pour into a greased baking dish and bake for 25-30 minutes.

Nutritional Values: Calories: 120, Protein: 3g, Carbs: 22g, Fat: 5g

Apple Cinnamon Energy Balls

Servings: 12 balls

Cooking Time: 10 minutes

Ingredients

1 cup rolled oats

1/2 cup dried apple, chopped

1/2 cup almond butter

1 tablespoon honey

1 teaspoon cinnamon

Instructions

1. Combine all ingredients in a bowl.
2. Roll mixture into balls and refrigerate for at least 30 minutes.

Nutritional Values: Calories: 130, Protein: 4g, Carbs: 20g, Fat: 6g

Coconut Milk Popsicles

Servings: 6

Cooking Time: 10 minutes + 4 hours freezing time

Ingredients

1 can full-fat coconut milk

1/4 cup honey

1 teaspoon vanilla extract

Optional: diced fruit or shredded coconut

Instructions

1. Mix coconut milk, honey, and vanilla extract.
2. Pour into popsicle molds.
3. Add diced fruit or shredded coconut if desired.
4. Freeze for at least 4 hours.

Nutritional Values: Calories: 150, Protein: 2g, Carbs: 14g, Fat: 10g

Dark Chocolate Dipped Strawberries

Servings: 8

Cooking Time: 10 minutes + 1 hour chilling time

Ingredients

1 cup dark chocolate chips

16 fresh strawberries

1 tablespoon coconut oil

Instructions

1. Melt chocolate chips with coconut oil in a microwave-safe bowl.
2. Dip strawberries into chocolate and place on a parchment-lined tray.
3. Chill for at least 1 hour.

Nutritional Values: Calories: 80, Protein: 1g, Carbs: 9g, Fat: 5g

8. 28-Day Meal Plan

Creating a 28-day meal plan with a daily calorie range of 500-1000 requires careful planning to ensure nutritional balance while staying within the calorie limits. This plan includes breakfast, lunch, dinner, and snacks for each day.

Week 1

Day 1

Breakfast: Error! Reference source not found. (200 calories)

Lunch: Error! Reference source not found.(300 calories)

Dinner: Error! Reference source not found. (200 calories)

Snack: Error! Reference source not found.(150 calories)

Total: 850 calories

Day 2

Breakfast: Error! Reference source not found. (160 calories)

Lunch: Error! Reference source not found. (180 calories)

Dinner: Error! Reference source not found. (250 calories)

Snack: Error! Reference source not found. (150 calories)

Total: 740 calories

Day 3

Breakfast: Error! Reference source not found. (250 calories)

Lunch: Error! Reference source not found. (250 calories)

Dinner: Error! Reference source not found. (300 calories)

Snack: Error! Reference source not found. (100 calories)

Total: 900 calories

Day 4

Breakfast: Error! Reference source not found. (180 calories)

Lunch: Error! Reference source not found. (300 calories)

Dinner: Error! Reference source not found. (300 calories)

Snack: Error! Reference source not found. (100 calories)

Total: 880 calories

Day 5

Breakfast: Error! Reference source not found. (150 calories)

Lunch: Error! Reference source not found. (140 calories)

Dinner: Error! Reference source not found. (250 calories)

Snack: Error! Reference source not found.(130 calories)

Total: 670 calories

Breakfast: Error! Reference source not found.(100 calories)

Lunch: Error! Reference source not found. (300 calories)

Dinner: Error! Reference source not found.(300 calories)

Snack: Error! Reference source not found. (120 calories)

Total: 820 calories

Day 7

Breakfast: Error! Reference source not found. (200 calories)

Lunch: Error! Reference source not found. (300 calories)

Dinner: Error! Reference source not found. (300 calories)

Snack: Error! Reference source not found. (100 calories)

Total: 900 calories

Week 2

Day 8

Breakfast: Error! Reference source not found. (160 calories)

Lunch: Error! Reference source not found. (250 calories)

Dinner: Error! Reference source not found. (300 calories)

Snack: Error! Reference source not found. (120 calories)

Total: 830 calories

Day 10

Breakfast: Error! Reference source not found.(180 calories)

Lunch: Error! Reference source not found.(180 calories)

Dinner: Error! Reference source not found. (250 calories)

Snack: Error! Reference source not found. (120 calories)

Total: 730 calories

Day 9

Breakfast: Error! Reference source not found. (150 calories)

Lunch: Error! Reference source not found.(250 calories)

Dinner: Error! Reference source not found. (300 calories)

Snack: Error! Reference source not found. (80 calories)

Total: 780 calories

Day 11

Breakfast: Error! Reference source not found. (250 calories)

Lunch: Error! Reference source not found. (160 calories)

Dinner: Error! Reference source not found. (250 calories)

Snack: Error! Reference source not found. (100 calories)

Total: 760 calories

Day 12

Breakfast: Error! Reference source not found. (220 calories)

Lunch: Error! Reference source not found. (320 calories)

Dinner: Error! Reference source not found. (280 calories)

Snack: Banana Oat Cookies (100 calories)

Total: 920 calories

Day 13

Breakfast: Error! Reference source not found. (160 calories)

Lunch: Error! Reference source not found. (220 calories)

Dinner: Error! Reference source not found. (350 calories)

Snack: Error! Reference source not found. (150 calories)

Total: 880 calories

Day 14

Breakfast: Error! Reference source not found. (150 calories)

Lunch: Error! Reference source not found. (250 calories)

Dinner: Error! Reference source not found. (250 calories)

Snack: Error! Reference source not found. (150 calories)

Total: 800 calories

Week 3

Day 15

Breakfast: Error! Reference source not found. (250 calories)

Lunch: Error! Reference source not found. (250 calories)

Dinner: Error! Reference source not found. (300 calories)

Snack: Error! Reference source not found. (120 calories)

Total: 920 calories

Day 16

Breakfast: Error! Reference source not found. (180 calories)

Lunch: Error! Reference source not found. (280 calories)

Dinner: Error! Reference source not found. (400 calories)

Snack: Error! Reference source not found.(130 calories)

Total: 980 calories

Day 17

Breakfast: Error! Reference source not found. (160 calories)

Lunch: Error! Reference source not found. (400 calories)

Dinner: Error! Reference source not found. (200 calories)

Snack: Error! Reference source not found. (100 calories)

Total: 860 calories

Day 18

Breakfast: Error! Reference source not found. (200 calories)

Lunch: Error! Reference source not found. (320 calories)

Dinner: Error! Reference source not found. (280 calories)

Snack: Error! Reference source not found. (80 calories)

Total: 880 calories

Day 19

Breakfast: Error! Reference source not found. (150 calories)

Lunch: Error! Reference source not found. (280 calories)

Dinner: Error! Reference source not found. (350 calories)

Snack: Error! Reference source not found. (100 calories)

Total: 870 calories

Day 20

Breakfast: Error! Reference source not found. (180 calories)

Lunch: Error! Reference source not found. (250 calories)

Dinner: Error! Reference source not found. (220 calories)

Snack: Error! Reference source not found. (120 calories)

Total: 770 calories

Day 21

Breakfast: Error! Reference source not found. (200 calories)

Lunch: Error! Reference source not found. (280 calories)

Dinner: Error! Reference source not found. (350 calories)

Snack: Error! Reference source not found. (150 calories)

Total: 980 calories

Week 4

Day 22

Breakfast: Error! Reference source not found. (200 calories)

Lunch: Error! Reference source not found. (300 calories)

Dinner: Error! Reference source not found. (300 calories)

Snack: Error! Reference source not found. (120 calories)

Total: 920 calories

Day 23

Breakfast: Error! Reference source not found. (150 calories)

Lunch: Error! Reference source not found. (300 calories)

Dinner: Error! Reference source not found. (250 calories)

Snack: Error! Reference source not found. (100 calories)

Total: 800 calories

Day 24

Breakfast: Error! Reference source not found. (200 calories)

Lunch: Error! Reference source not found. (300 calories)

Dinner: Error! Reference source not found. (250 calories)

Snack: Error! Reference source not found. (100 calories)

Total: 850 calories

Day 25

Breakfast: Error! Reference source not found. (250 calories)

Lunch: Error! Reference source not found. (300 calories)

Dinner: Error! Reference source not found. (250 calories)

Snack: Error! Reference source not found. (120 calories)

Total: 920 calories

Day 26

Breakfast: Error! Reference source not found. (200 calories)

Lunch: Error! Reference source not found. (150 calories)

Dinner: Error! Reference source not found. (400 calories)

Snack: Error! Reference source not found. (120 calories)

Total: 840 calories

Day 27

Breakfast: Error! Reference source not found. (200 calories)

Lunch: Error! Reference source not found. (350 calories)

Dinner: Error! Reference source not found. (300 calories)

Snack: Error! Reference source not found. (80 calories)

Total: 880 calories

Day 28

Breakfast: Error! Reference source not found. (180 calories)

Lunch: Error! Reference source not found. (280 calories)

Dinner: Cauliflower Fried Rice (200 calories)

Snack: Error! Reference source not found. (200 calories)

Total: 860 calories

This plan includes a balanced distribution of recipes, ensuring a variety of breakfast, lunch, dinner, and snack options while maintaining the calorie range between 500-1000 per day. Adjust portions as necessary to meet specific dietary needs.

Conclusion

Thank you for joining us on this journey through the "Easy Calorie Deficit Cookbook." We hope this collection of delicious, nutrient-rich recipes has inspired you to embrace a healthier lifestyle and empowered you to make mindful food choices. Maintaining a calorie deficit doesn't have to mean sacrificing flavor or satisfaction, and we trust that the meals in this book have proven just that.

Throughout these pages, we've explored the essentials of balanced eating, provided you with practical tools and techniques for healthy cooking, and offered a wide array of recipes to keep your palate excited and your body nourished. From wholesome breakfasts and satisfying lunches to nutritious dinners, smart snacks, and guilt-free desserts, you've now got a wealth of options to support your weight loss goals while enjoying every bite.

Remember, achieving and maintaining a healthy weight is a marathon, not a sprint. It's about making sustainable changes that fit into your lifestyle and become part of your daily routine. The recipes and tips provided in this book are designed to be flexible and adaptable, allowing you to personalize your approach to healthy eating.

Measurement and Conversions

CUPS	OZ	G	TBSP	TSP	ML
1	8	225	16	48	250
3/4	6	170	12	36	175
2/3	5	140	11	32	150
1/2	4	115	8	24	125
1/3	3	70	5	16	70
1/4	2	60	4	12	60
1/8	1	30	2	6	30
1/16	1/2	15	1	3	15

250°F	300°F	325°F	350°F	400°F	450°F
120°C	150°F	160°C	175°C	200°C	230°C

About the Author

Abibat Oladunjoye is a passionate advocate for healthy living and an accomplished culinary expert dedicated to making nutritious eating both enjoyable and accessible. With years of experience in the kitchen and a deep understanding of nutrition, Abibat has crafted the "Easy Calorie Deficit Cookbook" to help readers achieve their weight loss goals without sacrificing taste or satisfaction.

Recipe Index